Eat Healthy,

Be Healthy

Eat Healthy,
Be Healthy

Zahra Yasmin Soltanian

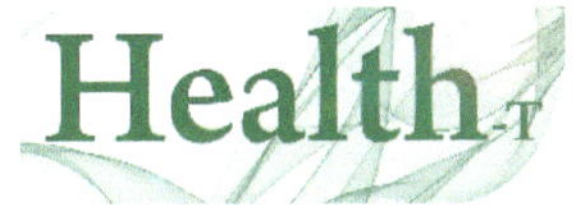

Health-T Publication

This edition first published in 2020

ISBN 978-0-473-53986-3 (paperback)

ISBN 978-0-473-53987-0 (kindle)

A catalogue record for this book is available from the National Library of New Zealand.

Published by Health-T Publication, Auckland

Contents

Introduction

I once heard a family member ask: How much is your body and health worth to you? Almost everyone would answer that their body and health is priceless and probably one of the most important things that an individual owns. Neglecting one's well-being and developing unhealthy habits, quickly leads to the breakdown and deterioration of health. Overtime, the deterioration of health could result in various different ailments and conditions that lower an individual's quality of life and their lifespan.

It is never too late to improve one's physical and mental health by getting rid of unhealthy habits and adopting new beneficial ones. One of the most important factors for an individual's health is their eating habits and what they put into their bodies. Eating foods that are high in nutritional value and low in calories are essential in staying healthy and maintaining a healthy weight. Eating healthy and keeping to a healthy weight has the added benefit of looking good. Eating in a way that allows the body to function in the best possible way and stay healthy longer requires a delicate balance of getting the right nutrients and the right amount of energy.

Each person's needs are different and a diet plan should be based on an individual's goals and needs. For, example, it is important for people to recognise that two people that are of different size, genetics and sex do not have the same daily dietary intake requirements in order to maintain a healthy weight range. For a person to maintain their healthy weight, they need to consume the same amount of nutritional calories that their body uses during the day. If a person consumes more than their body needs, the body usually stores it as excess weight in the form of fat. If a person consumes less than what their body uses on a daily basis, the body uses what it already has to produce the energy it needs to function. So if the person has excess fat storage, the body tends to it to produce the energy it needs, resulting in weight loss. If a person is intending to lose weight they must consume fewer calories than their body uses until they achieve their desired weight. Size, sex and genetics can all affect the amount of energy that a person requires and needs to get through food consumption to stay healthy. For example, a 153cm female does not need as much calories as a 180cm tall male to maintain a healthy body weight.

Changing unhealthy habits to healthy ones requires fundamental changes both in terms of a person's habits as well as their thinking. In regards to food, it isn't as simple to eat healthy and low calorie food if unhealthy eating habits and tastes are not replaced with healthy ones. It is important that a person changes their tastes so as to not crave unhealthy, high calorie foods. This change must be permanent so that there is no relapse to an unhealthy lifestyle. In order to achieve the long-term goal of staying healthy through a beneficial diet plan, a person needs to change their eating habits and thinking about food. Such an adjustment might take a period of time but through consistency a person's taste will eventually change towards preferring the healthier food options. For example, if a person is used to sweetened food, removing sugar and sweet food will be difficult at the beginning. They might find the new food bland and unappetising. However, as the person consistently keeps to a low sugar diet they will become accustomed and even aversive to excessively sweetened foods. They tend to discover tastes that were usually masked by sugar or excessive salt.

If a person is used to eating in a way that results in unhealthy weight gains then the only way to change their habit is through adopting healthy practices and a new way of thinking. A person has to remind themselves that food serves the purpose of giving the body the energy it requires to function. If an individual is putting on unhealthy weight then they are eating more than the energy that their body needs. This does not mean that people should not enjoy eating, it only means that food can be enjoyed without exceeding the amount of calories required to maintain a healthy weight.

As a parent a person might be interested in making sure that their kids become accustomed to good eating habits and the health benefits that go with it. In fact, it is best to start children with healthy eating habits. Many parents make the mistake of thinking it is ok to leave their children to indulge in unhealthy eating habits until they grow up. However, such a mistaken belief results in childhood health issues that can then affect their adulthood. In addition, if children are not given the right guidance at earlier stages of their life, they will grow up with habits that are hard to give up as adults. For example, becoming used to eating unhealthy foods with flavour enhancers could destroy the bodies' natural ability to regulate what and how much they should eat. Their taste buds might develop to only like very sweet, salty or oily food. It is expected from a parent that they should never allow their children to smoke. The fact, that they are children is even more the reason to stop them from smoking due to the harm it can cause on a short-term and long-term basis. Similarly, just like any other healthy versus unhealthy habits, parents should teach their children how to eat healthy so that their taste develops accordingly into adulthood.

If you are reading this book, it means you are interested in having a healthy eating habit. As mentioned before, a healthy diet is one that provides a person with various different nutrients good for the health and the right amount, not more, energy for the body to function. A nutrient-calorie balanced diet can be achieved by adding different ingredients from different food groups to a meal to obtain vital minerals and vitamins while still keeping that meal low in calories. The energy contained in foods which is used by the body to function is calculated through the unit of measurement known as nutritional calories (a nutritional calorie is equivalent to 1 kilocalorie as a unit of energy). If you are the type who gets bored with eating the same foods then you can swap ingredients with each meal, keeping it both low calorie and nutritious.

Another factor to take into consideration when trying to keep healthy and maintain a healthy weight is the way in which food is cooked. For example, if a person is frying every meal with oil (even healthy ones like olive oil), this will add to their overall calorie intake. Some better and healthier options for preparing meals can include steam cooking, boiling or roasting in the oven. Electricity costs can be kept to a minimal by cooking in small bench-top ovens. A small bench-top oven can easily cook for up to six people.

Many people find it difficult to lose or maintain weight even though they do not eat much food. In many cases, the problem has nothing to do with quantity of food. Different food ingredients vary in terms of the calories they contain per volume. A hundred gram of cashew nuts has about 550 to 560 calories whereas the same volume of lettuce (100 grams) has about 15 calories. This means that to get the same calories of 100 grams of cashew nuts a person would have to eat about 3700 grams (3.7 kg) of lettuce. In order to lose weight or maintain a healthy weight range a person has to prepare meals in a way that considers calories contained in each ingredient.

In this book I have compiled a number of tasty recipes for low calorie dishes that are also high in nutrients to help individuals achieve the right balance of consuming what the body needs while maintaining a healthy weight. Many of the meals in this book are made with a variety of spices (such as ginger and chilli) that both add to the taste and provide healthy nutrients. I have divided the book into sections that categorise each recipe into dishes that are plant-based (containing no animal products or dairy), seafood meals, egg based dishes, chicken dishes and meals that have red meat as their main ingredients.

This book is not an exhaustive list of low calorie and healthy recipes. It is only intended to give an idea about different ways healthy food ingredients can be combined to be both low calorie and tasty. An individual can pick from a variety of the recipes provided in this book to organise their daily intake in accordance to their appropriate calorie and nutrient needs. Any three dishes made with the recipes in this book would equal to only about a 1000 calories or less. It is important for an individual to calculate their overall needed calorie intake based on their physical requirements and goals through appropriate tools then use the recipes and information contained in this book to achieve the desired weight.

The serving size of each recipe is for one person. However, if the intention is to cook for more than one person then each ingredient can be proportionally increased. For example, if for one person the recipe requires 200 grams of mushrooms then for two that should be doubled to 400 grams and for three to 600 grams and so on. Also, as stated above, different people have different calorie requirements. For that reason, the amount of each of the ingredients in the recipes can be adjusted to satisfy individual calorie needs (for example, increased for more calorie needs). Just make sure to calculate and include as your daily intake, calories from other foods, such as fruits, consumed in addition to meals made with these recipes.

Disclaimer

What you read in this book and the recipes provided are based on my own personal research and weight loss journey. It is intended to provide some information and a few tips on how to maintain weight while receiving the nutrients needed for physical health. For precise advice and a diet plan suited on an individual level, I recommend seeking the advice of a health practitioner or registered dietician.

1　Plant-Based Dishes

Dishes that contain plant-based ingredients
(No animal products or dairy)

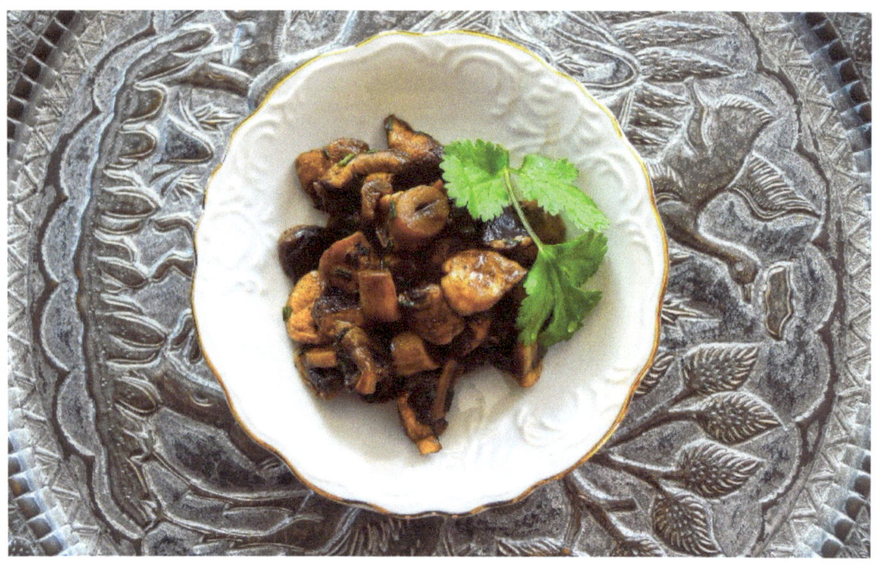

Chive Mushrooms

Calories: ~110 (nutritional calories)

Serving size: 1 Person

Ingredients:

- 200 Grams button mushrooms

- 1 Teaspoon extra virgin olive oil (for cooking)

- ¼ Teaspoon onion powder

- 1 Teaspoon chives

- ½ Teaspoon crushed garlic

- Salt and pepper to season

- Coriander to garnish

Preparation:

1. Turn on oven temperature to 200 degrees Celsius (392 degrees Fahrenheit).

2. Wash the mushrooms thoroughly removing any soil.

3. Chop mushrooms into half- length sizes.

4. Season the mushrooms with onion powder, chives, garlic, salt and pepper.

5. Place the mushrooms on an oven tray and cover the tray with foil. This will steam the mushrooms without drying them out.

6. Roast the mushrooms for 30 minutes until cooked.

7. Garnish with coriander.

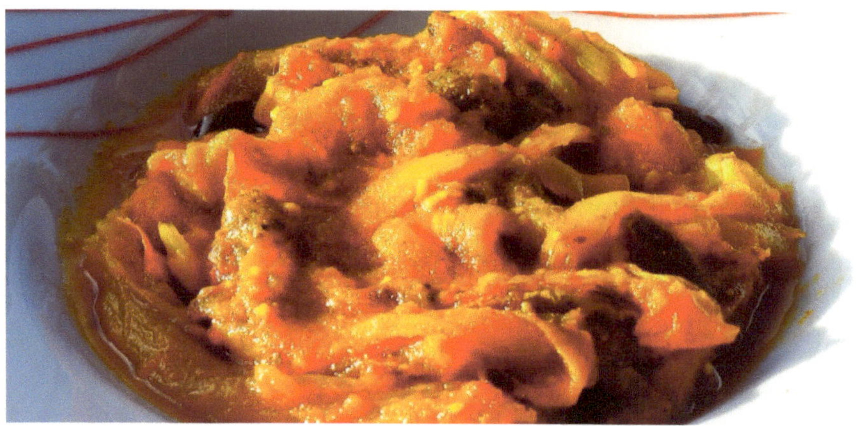

Eggplant Stew

Calories: ~ 144 (nutritional calories)

Serving size: 1 Person

Ingredients:

- 200 Grams (one cup) eggplant

- 1 Medium sized tomato

- 1 Small onion

- 1 Tablespoon 100 percent tomato paste (no sugar)

- ½ Teaspoon turmeric

- ½ Teaspoon crushed garlic

- Salt and pepper to season

Preparation:

1. Turn on oven temperature to 200 degrees Celsius (392 degrees Fahrenheit).

2. Wash and cut the eggplants and tomatoes lengthwise in half. Do not remove the stem of the eggplant.

3. Chop the onions in thin slices, lengthwise.

4. Chop the tomatoes into quarters.

5. Place all the vegetables on an oven tray.

6. Roast in the oven for 1 hour or until the eggplants are soft.

7. Scoop out the eggplant by holding onto the stem. Alternatively, if you prefer the eggplant with the skin, chop the eggplant into chunky pieces.

8. Transfer to a pan with the tomatoes and onions.

9. Add the tomato paste, turmeric, salt, pepper and garlic.

10. Cook the vegetables a further 10 minutes until all the flavours are blended into the dish.

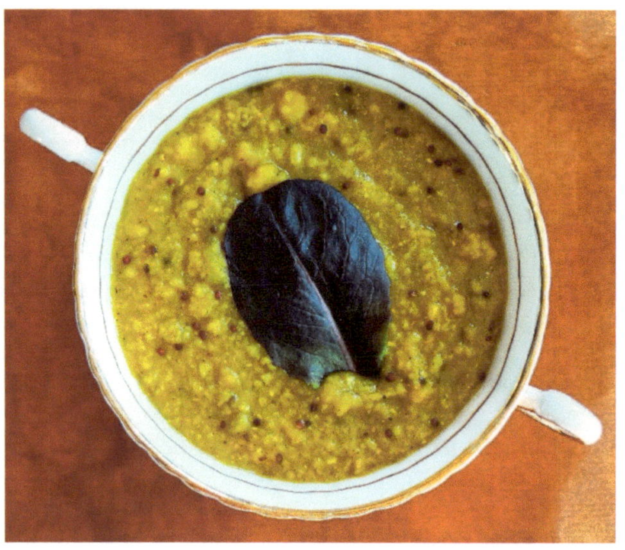

Dhal Soup

Calories: ~220 (nutritional calories)

Serving size: 1 Person

Ingredients:

- 50 Grams yellow split peas

- 1 Small onion

- ¼ Teaspoon turmeric

- 1 Teaspoon garlic chives

- ¼ Teaspoon cinnamon

- ¼ Teaspoon black mustard seeds

- ¼ Teaspoon cumin

- ¼ Teaspoon coriander powder

- Salt and pepper to season

Preparation:

1. Soak the yellow split peas the night before. This reduces the cooking time if you using a pressure cooker. If you are cooking in a pressure cooker, this step is not necessary.

2. Pour the yellow split peas in the pressure cooker.

3. Chop onions into small pieces.

4. Add the chopped onions, garlic chives, cinnamon, mustard seeds, cumin and coriander powder to the yellow split pea.

5. Add salt and pepper to taste.

6. Cover the lentils with enough water to soak the lentils.

7. Cook for about 10 minutes (if using a pressure cooker) or until the lentils are soft.

8. With a hand blender, blend the mixture until pureed to the consistency of smooth paste.

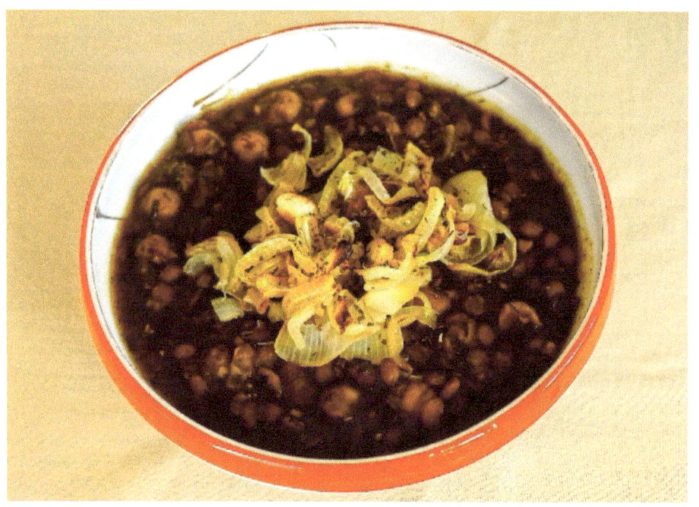

Aash soup

Calories: ~233 (nutritional calories)

Serving size: 1 Person

Ingredients:

- 20 Grams chickpeas
- 20 Grams kidney beans
- 20 Grams black-eyed beans
- 20 Grams brown lentils
- 1 Teaspoon chives
- 1 Teaspoon dill
- ¼ Teaspoon turmeric
- ¼ Teaspoon mint
- 1 Small onion
- Salt and pepper to season

Preparation:

1. Soak the chickpeas, kidney beans, black eyed beans and brown lentils over night for a faster cooking time.

2. Place chickpeas, kidney beans, black-eyed beans, brown lentils in a pressure cooker.

3. Add chives, dill and turmeric.

4. Add salt and pepper to taste.

5. Add water to soak the mixture.

6. Cook until the lentils and legumes are soft.

7. Cut one small onion lengthwise into thin slices.

8. Roast the onions in an oven until golden brown.

9. Pour the soup mixture into a bowl.

10. Garnish with roasted onions and mint.

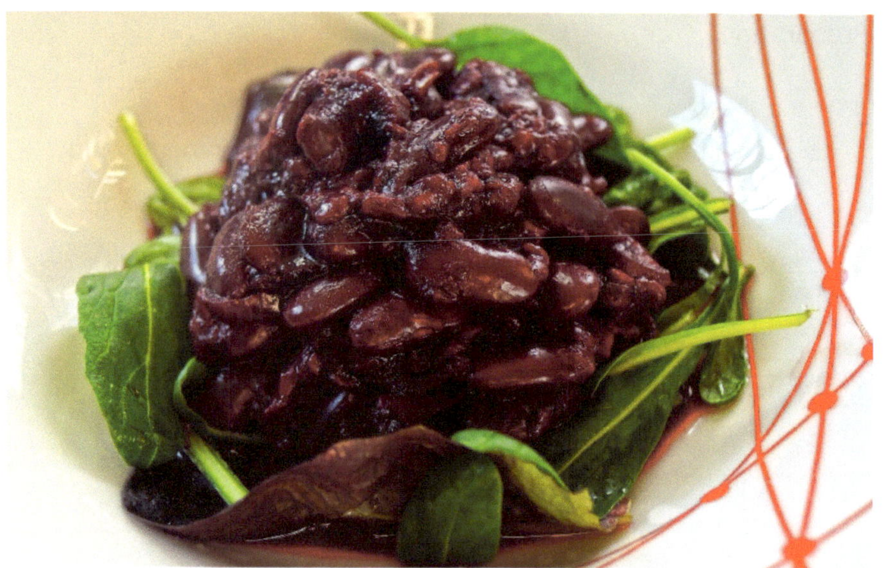

Boysenberry Beans

Calories: ~235 (nutritional calories)

Serving size: 1 Person

Ingredients:

- 50 Grams red kidney beans

- 50 Grams boysenberries

- 1 Small onion

- Salt and pepper to season

- 50 Grams mixed salad leaves (Oaks, batavia, butter, cos, beet, chard, spinach and mibuna leaves)

Preparation:

1. Pre-soak the kidney beans overnight for faster cooking time.

2. Chop one small onion into small pieces.

3. Place the kidney beans, chopped onions and boysenberries into a pressure cooker.

4. Level the beans with enough water to cover the mixture.

5. Add salt and pepper to season.

6. Cook until the beans are soft.

7. Stir the kidney beans, onions and boysenberries after taking out of the pressure cooker to mix in the sauce.

8. Serve the beans with a base of assorted salad leaves.

2 Seafood Dishes

Dishes with fish or other seafood as the main ingredient

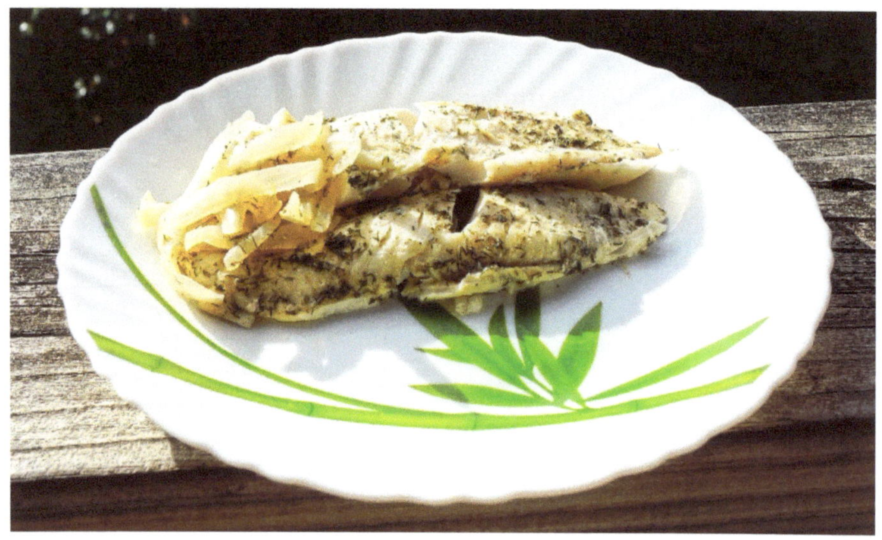

Dill Lemon Fish

Calories: ~188 (nutritional calories)

Serving size: 1 Person

Ingredients:

- 150 Grams tarakihi fish (any white fish can be used)
- 1 Small onion
- Juice of one lemon
- ¼ Teaspoon cumin
- 1 Teaspoon dried dill
- Salt and pepper to season

Preparation:

1. Turn oven on to 200 degrees Celsius (392 degrees Fahrenheit).

2. Season the fish with lemon juice, dill, salt and pepper.

3. Wrap the seasoned fish with the chopped onions in some foil.

4. Place in the oven for 30 minutes.

5. Cook until the fish is tender.

6. Serve in a dish.

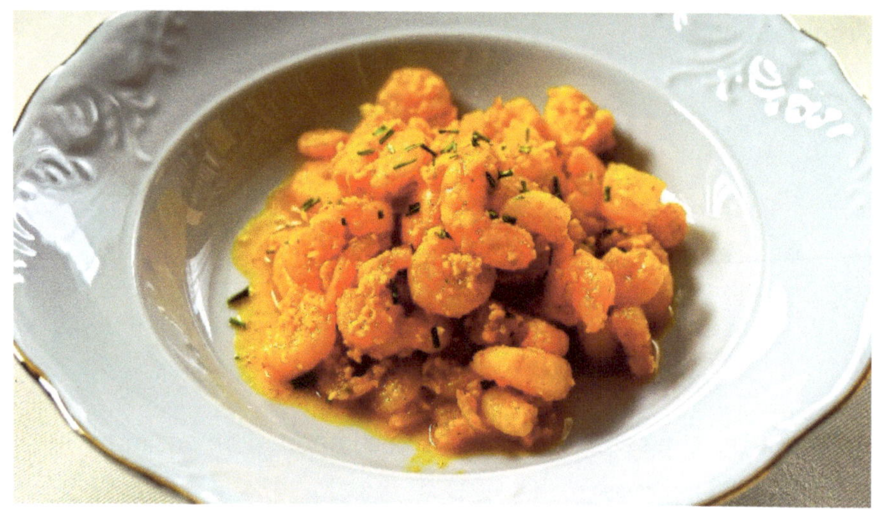

Kaffir Lime Orange Shrimps

Calories: ~223 (nutritional calories)

Serving size: 1 Person

Ingredients:

- 150 Grams shrimps

- 1 Small onion

- Juice of one kaffir lime

- Orange rind to taste

- ½ Teaspoon crushed ginger

- ½ Teaspoon crushed garlic

- ½ Teaspoon chilli powder

- ½ Teaspoon turmeric

- Salt and pepper to season

Preparation:

1. Wash the shrimps well. Remove any shells (if you prefer).

2. Chop one onion into small pieces.

3. Grate the rind of one orange. Set aside.

4. Boil the shrimps and onions for 15 minutes.

5. Transfer to a pan.

6. Add the juice of kaffir lime, orange rind, crushed ginger, crushed garlic, chilli powder and turmeric.

7. Add salt and pepper to taste.

8. Sauté the shrimps with the flavours for a further five minutes.

9. Garnish with dried chives.

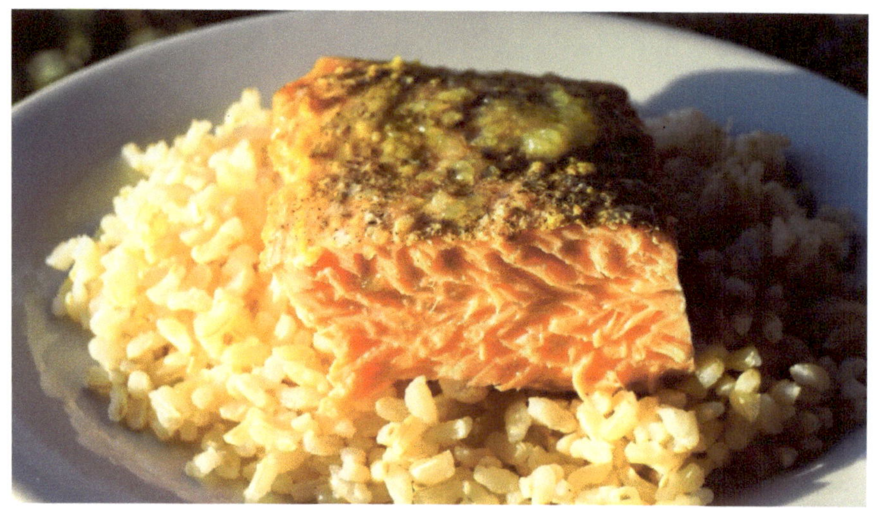

Lime Salmon with Brown Rice

Calories: ~228 (nutritional calories)

Serving size: 1 Person

Ingredients:

- 100 Grams salmon

- 1 Lime

- Salt and pepper to season

- 50 Grams wholegrain brown rice

Preparation:

1. Sprinkle salt and pepper over the salmon (be generous with the pepper).

2. Grate the rind of one lime and rub zest onto the salmon.

3. Wrap salmon with aluminium foil and leave to cook in the oven at a temperature of 200 degrees Celsius (392 degrees Fahrenheit).

4. Pour rice into a pot with enough water to cover the rice. Add more water as needed.

5. Cook rice for about 20 minutes or until cooked.

6. Drain the rice of excess water.

7. Unwrap salmon and sprinkle the juice of one lime over the salmon and serve with rice

3   Egg Dishes

Dishes with egg as the main ingredient

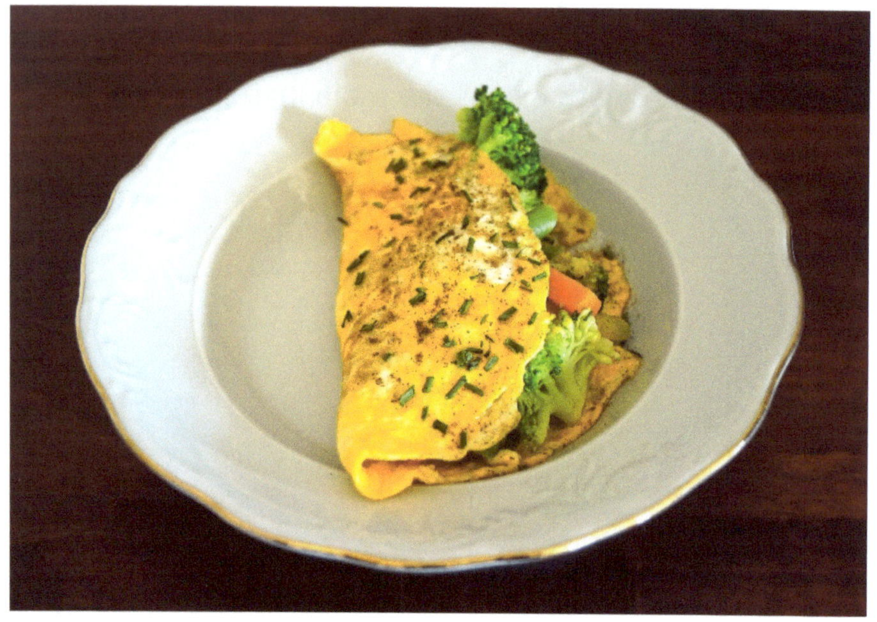

Vegetable Egg Wrap

Calories: ~154 (nutritional calories)

Serving size: 1 Person

Ingredients:

- 1 Chicken egg (size 7)

- 50 Grams of mixed vegetables (broccoli, carrots, green beans, butter beans, capsicum)

- ½ Teaspoon chives

- Salt and pepper to season

- 1 Teaspoon extra virgin olive oil (for cooking)

Preparation:

1. Heat the olive oil in a small frying pan.

2. Scramble one chicken egg and pour into the oil, spreading it out around the pan.

3. Season the eggs with salt, chives and pepper. Remove from heat once the eggs are cooked.

4. Boil the vegetables until cooked.

5. Place the vegetables on one half of the eggs.

6. Flip the other half of the egg over to cover the vegetables.

7. Garnish with more chives.

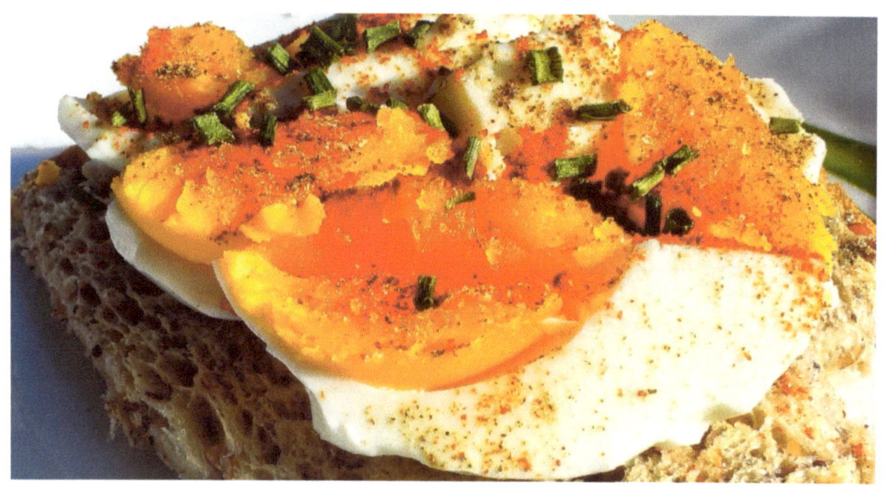

Chilli Egg and Toast

Calories: ~165 (nutritional calories)

Serving size: 1 Person

Ingredients:

- 1 Chicken egg (size 7)

- 1 Slice high protein wholegrain bread (this is dependent on the bread. The brand used in this recipe contains 82.5 nutritional calories for one slice)

- ½ Teaspoon chives

- Chilli powder to season

- Salt and pepper to season

Preparation:

1. Boil one chicken egg until the yoke is hard (or if you like it runny, reduce the boiling time).

2. Remove eggshell and cut into quarters.

3. Season the egg with chives, chilli powder, salt and pepper.

4.   Place the egg quarters on 1 slice of wholegrain bread and serve.

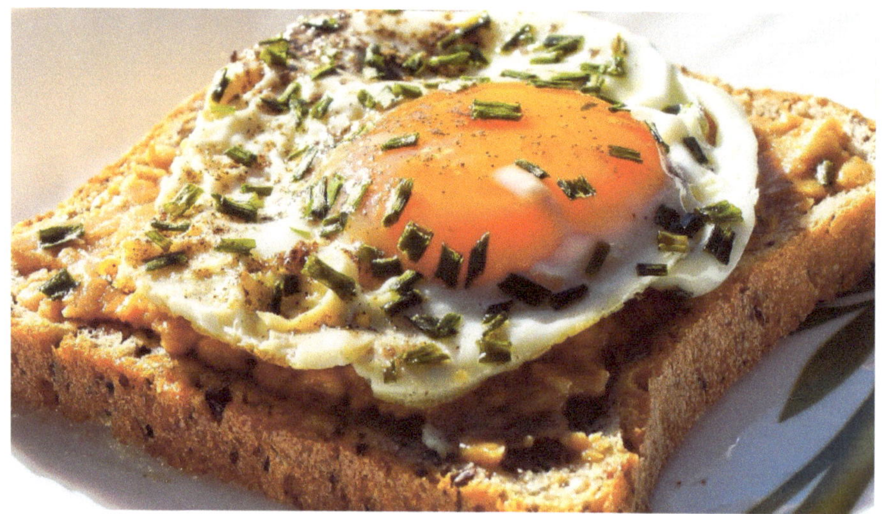

Egg, Peanut Butter and Toast

Calories: ~340 (nutritional calories)

Serving size: 1 Person

Ingredients:

- 1 Chicken egg (size 7)

- 1 Slice high protein wholegrain bread (this is dependent on the bread. The brand used in this recipe contains 82.5 nutritional calories for one slice)

- ½ Teaspoon chives

- 1 Tablespoon peanut butter

- Salt and pepper to season

- 1 Teaspoon extra virgin olive oil (for cooking)

Preparation:

1. Heat a teaspoon of olive oil in a pan.

2. Crack an egg into the pan.

3. Fry the egg until the whites are done (or more if you prefer the yoke to be cooked as well).

4. Season the egg with salt, pepper and chives.

5. Place the egg on 1 slice of bread with peanut butter and serve. (This recipe is adjusted (addition of peanut butter and oil) for those who may have different calorie requirements for weight maintenance.)

The egg, peanut butter and toast meal packs a lot of energy and is high calories. It is best suited as an energy food and is best for breakfast.

4   Chicken Dishes

Dishes with chicken as the main ingredient

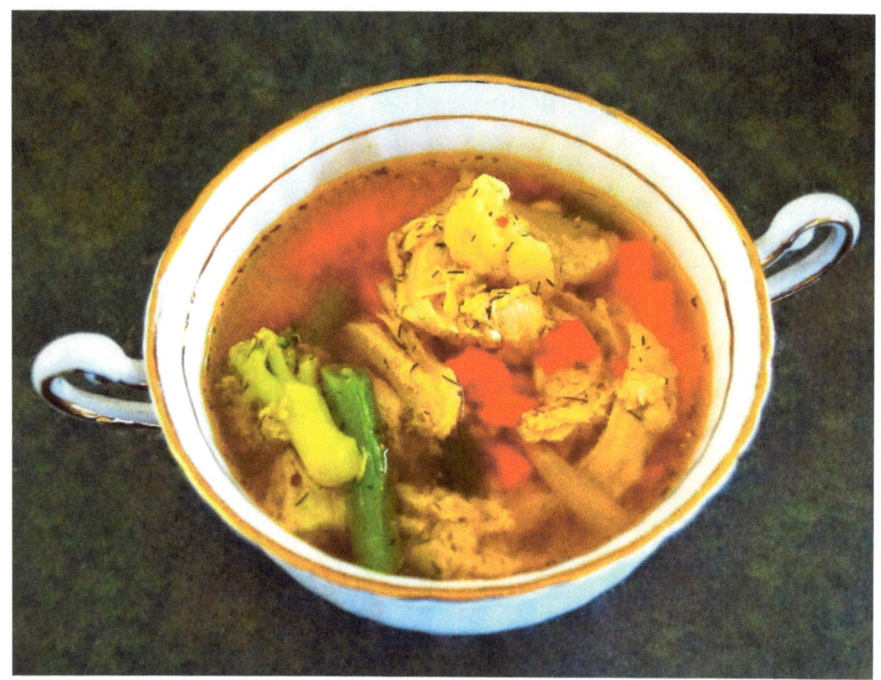

Chicken Soup

Calories: ~174 (nutritional calories)

Serving size: 1 Person

Ingredients:

- 50 Grams of chicken breasts

- 1 Chicken egg (size 7)

- 50 Grams of mixed vegetables (butter beans, green beans, cauliflower, capsicum and carrots)

- Salt and pepper to season

Preparation:

1. Chop the chicken breasts into small pieces.

2. Put the chicken pieces and vegetables into a pot.

3. Add enough water to cover the mixture.

4. Season with salt and pepper and boil for 10 minutes.

5. Scramble one chicken egg and pour the egg slowly into the pot while it is boiling. The egg will break and produce thin strands.

6. Turn off the heat and let the soup simmer until ready to serve.

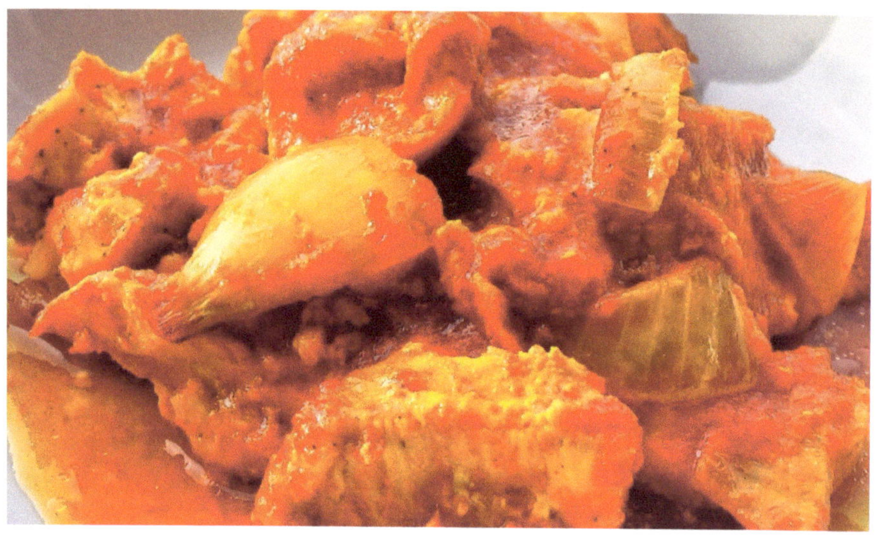

Saffron Chicken

Calories: ~240 (nutritional calories)

Serving size: 1 Person

Ingredients:

- 100 Grams of chicken breasts

- 1 Small onion

- 1 Tablespoon 100 percent tomato paste (no sugar)

- ½ Teaspoon turmeric

- ¼ Teaspoon saffron

- Salt and pepper to season

Preparation:

1. Turn oven on to 200 degrees Celsius (392 degrees Fahrenheit).

2. Chop the chicken into small cube size pieces.

3. Place them in an oven dish.

4. Season the chicken pieces with tomato paste, turmeric, saffron, salt and pepper.

5. Add chopped onions to the chicken.

6. Cover the dish with foil or other appropriate lid. This allows the chicken to cook in its own juices without drying out.

7. Place in the oven for 1 hour or until the chicken is tender.

8. Serve on a dish.

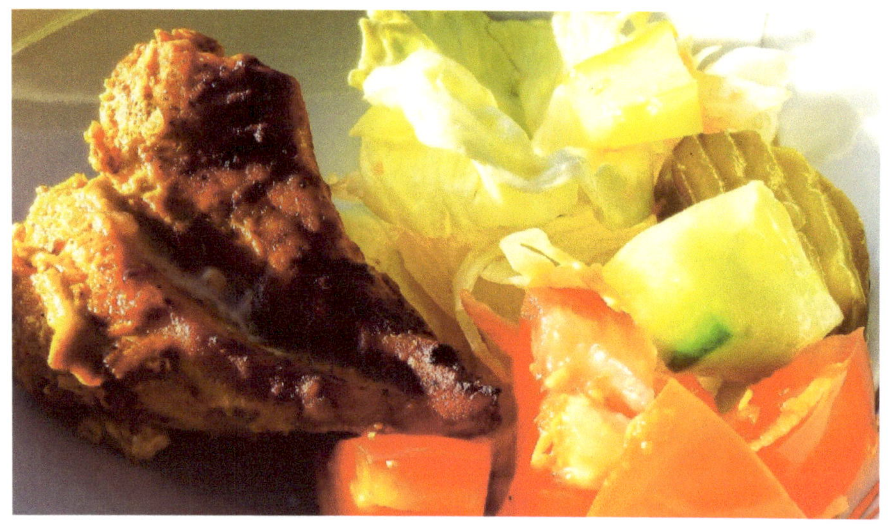

Tandoori Flavoured Chicken

Calories: ~238 (nutritional calories)

Serving size: 1 Person

Ingredients:

- 100 Grams of chicken breasts

- 1 Teaspoon tandoori powder

- 1 Tablespoon 100 percent tomato paste (no sugar)

- ½ Teaspoon turmeric

- Salt and pepper to season

- Salad: 50 grams lettuce, ½ tomato and 30 grams sliced gherkins

Preparation:

1. Turn oven on to 200 degrees Celsius (392 degrees Fahrenheit).

2. Chop the chicken into small pieces.

3. Place them in an oven dish.

4. Season the chicken pieces with tomato paste, turmeric, tandoori powder, salt and pepper.

5. Cover the dish with foil or other appropriate lid.

6. Place in the oven for 1 hour or until the chicken is tender.

7. Serve the chicken accompanied with salad.

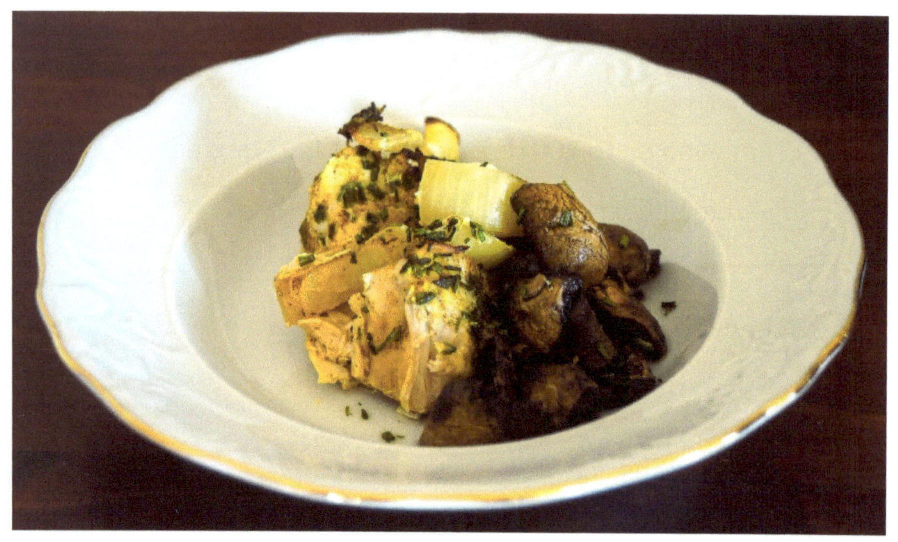

Mushroom Chicken

Calories: ~220 (nutritional calories)

Serving size: 1 Person

Ingredients:

- 100 Grams of chicken breasts
- 50 Grams button mushrooms
- ½ Small onion
- ½ Teaspoon turmeric
- ½ Teaspoon chives
- Salt and pepper to season

Preparation:

1. Turn oven on to 200 degrees Celsius (392 degrees Fahrenheit).

2. Chop the chicken into small cube size pieces.

3. Place them in an oven dish.

4. Add the chopped onions and button mushrooms.

5. Season the chicken pieces, onions and mushrooms with turmeric, chives, salt and pepper.

6. Cover the dish with foil or other appropriate lid.

7. Place in the oven for 1 hour or until the chicken is tender.

8. Place the chicken on a serving plate and garnish with chives.

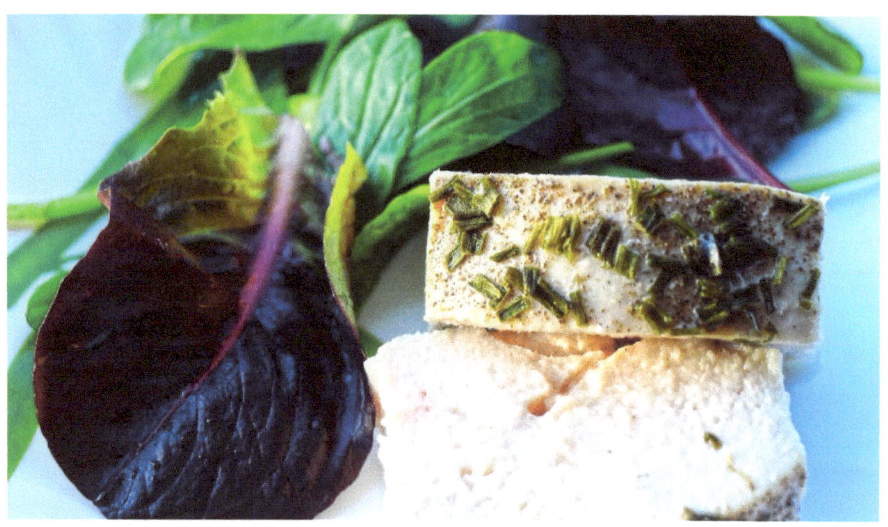

Boiled Chicken and Vegetable Leaves

Calories: ~180 (nutritional calories)

Serving size: 1 Person

Ingredients:

- 100 Grams of chicken breasts

- 1 Teaspoon chives

- 50 Grams of mixed salad leaves (Oaks, batavia, butter, cos, beet, chard, spinach and mibuna leaves)

- Salt and pepper to season

Preparation:

1. Cut the chicken into two pieces.

2. Place them in an oven dish.

3. Season the chicken pieces with chives, salt and pepper.

4. Cover the dish with foil.

5. Place in the oven for 1 hour or until the chicken is tender.

6. Serve with an assortment of salad leaves.

4 Red Meat Dishes

Dishes with red meat as the main ingredient

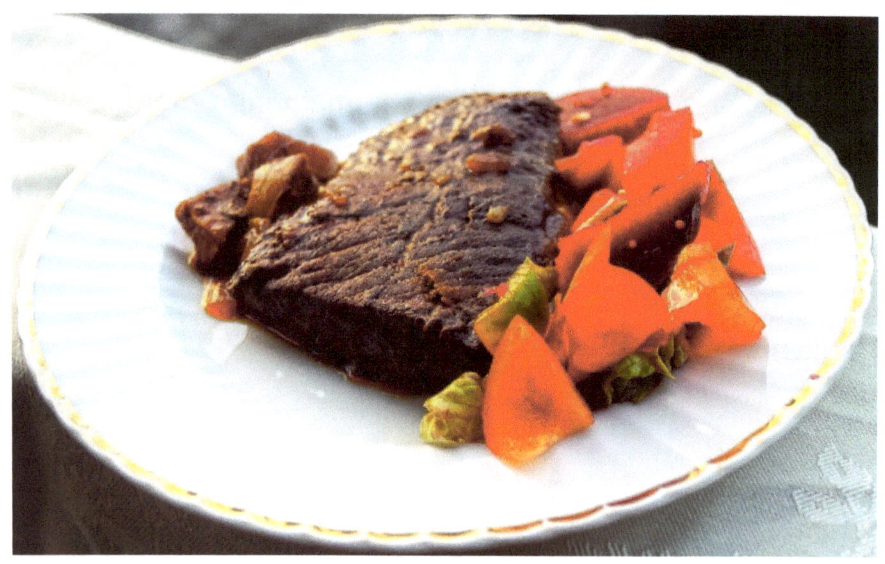

Steak with Quince Sauce

Calories: ~300 (nutritional calories)

Serving size: 1 Person

Ingredients:

- 150 Grams beef steak (calories might be different depending on the type of meat you use)
- 50 Grams chopped fresh quince
- 1 Teaspoon 100 percent tomato paste (no sugar)
- 1 Small onion
- ½ Teaspoon turmeric
- Salt and pepper to season
- 2 Tablespoons lemon juice

Preparation:

1. Turn oven on to 200 degrees Celsius (392 degrees Fahrenheit).

2. Place the steak and quince in an oven dish.

3. Season the steak and quince with salt, pepper, turmeric, and tomato paste and lemon juice.

4. Cover the dish with some foil.

5. Leave to cook until the steak is prepared to your liking.

6. You can complement your meal with a nutritious salad.

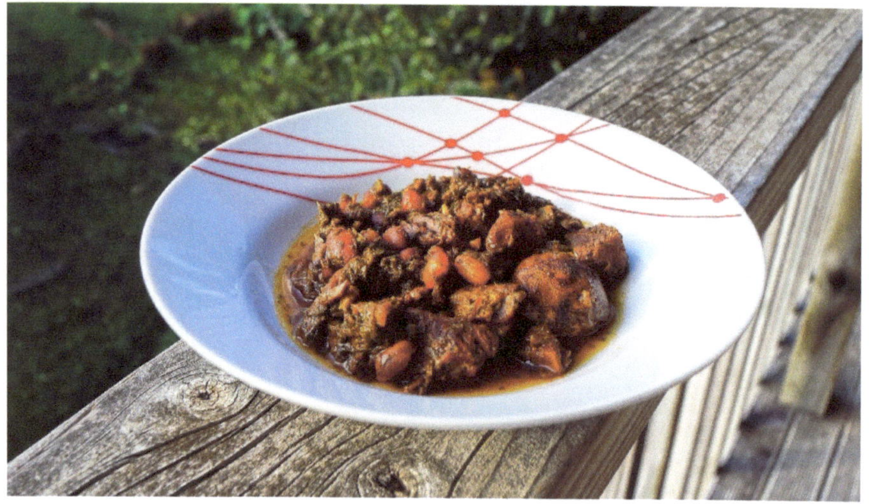

Ghormeh Sabzi (Low Calorie Version)

Calories: ~330 (nutritional calories)

Serving size: 1 Person

Ingredients:

- 50 Grams diced lean lamb pieces
- 1 Dried lime
- 1 Small onion
- 25 Grams red kidney beans
- 100 Grams mixed herbs (Parsley, coriander and spring onions)
- 1 Tablespoon fenugreek leaves
- 1 Tablespoon turmeric
- Salt and pepper to season

Preparation:

1. Place all the ingredients in a pressure cooker.

2. Add enough water to cover the meat.

3. Leave to cook until ready. Although this is not the traditional way of preparing this meal, it is a lower calorie, healthier option.

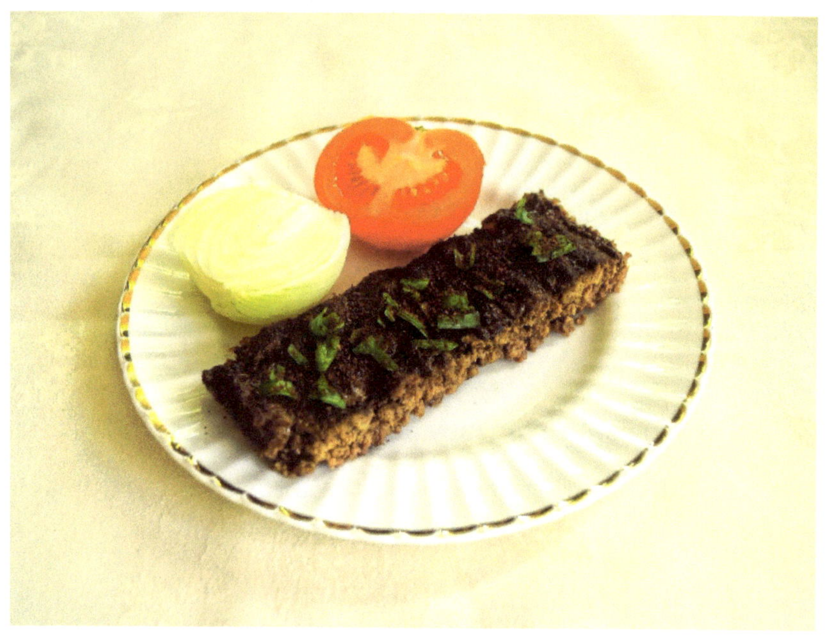

Mince Oven Kebabs

Calories: ~ 205 (nutritional calories)

Serving size: 1 Person

Ingredients:

- 50 Grams lean beef minced
- ½ Small onion and ½ tomato
- ½ Teaspoon turmeric and cumin
- 1 Tablespoon crushed garlic
- 1 Tablespoon sumac
- 1 Tablespoon coriander
- Salt and pepper to season

Preparation:

1. Turn oven on to 200 degrees Celsius (392 degrees Fahrenheit).

2. Combine minced beef with salt, pepper, turmeric, cumin and garlic until well mixed.

3. Spread and flatten the mixture out in a roasting tray.

4. Cook in the oven until the meat is done.

5. Cut the meat into long rectangular pieces as shown in the picture above.

6. Sprinkle sumac and garnish with coriander.

7. Serve the kebabs with onions and tomatoes.

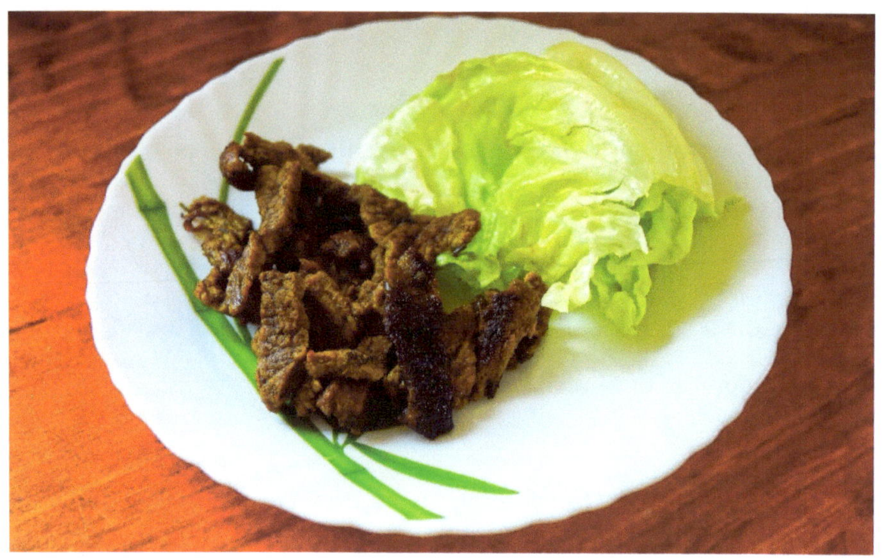

Flavoured Beef Strips with Lettuce

Calories: ~320 (nutritional calories)

Serving size: 1 Person

Ingredients:

- 100 Grams beef strips
- 1 Teaspoon extra virgin olive oil (for cooking)
- 1 Tablespoon chopped chives
- 50 Grams of lettuce
- Salt and pepper to season

Preparation:

1.   Heat olive oil in a pan.

2.   Fry the beef strips until golden brown.

3.   Add salt, pepper and chives.

4.   Serve the beef strips with some crunchy lettuce.

To reduce the calories, instead of frying the beef strips with oil, cook without olive oil in the oven.

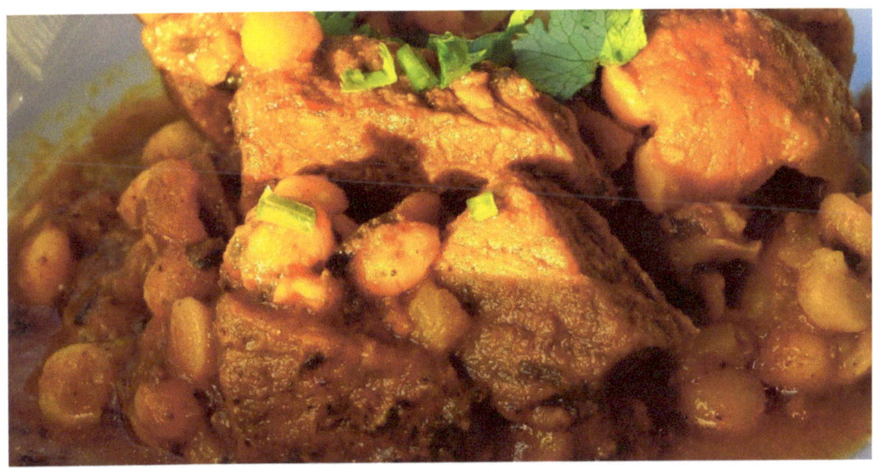

Khoresh Gheymeh

Calories: ~314 (nutritional calories)

Serving size: 1 Person

Ingredients:

- 50 Grams diced beef or lamb

- One small onion

- 30 Grams yellow split peas

- 1 Tablespoon 100 percent tomato paste (no sugar)

- 1 Dried lime

- ½ Teaspoon turmeric

- ½ Teaspoon cinnamon

- Salt and pepper

- Coriander for garnish

Preparation:

1. In a bowl, season the meat with all the spices.

2. Chop the onions and add to the meat.

3. Add the crushed dried lime, tomato paste and yellow split peas and place in a pressure cooker.

4. Add enough water to cover the meat.

5. Leave to cook until meat is tender.

6. Place the meat in a serving bowl and garnish with coriander.

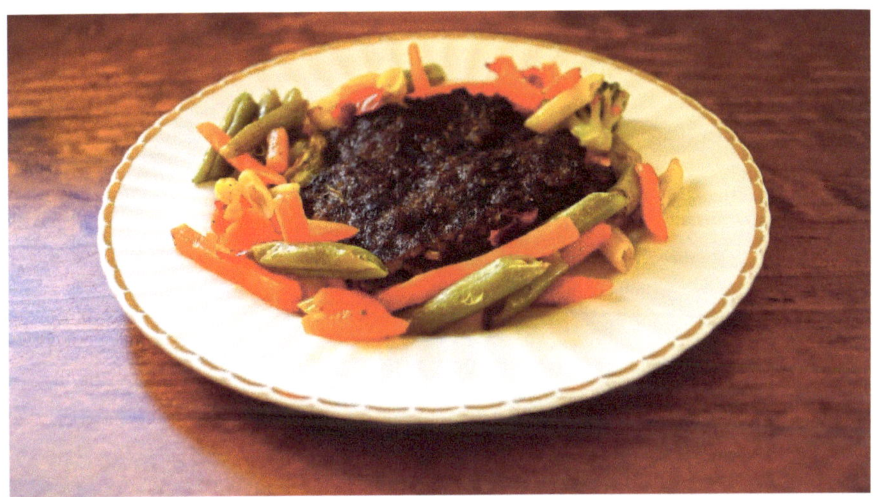

Mince Kebab

Calories: ~ 235 (nutritional calories)

Serving size: 1 Person

Ingredients:

- 50 Grams lean beef minced

- ½ Small onion

- ½ Teaspoon turmeric

- ½ Teaspoon cinnamon

- 1 Tablespoon chopped chives

- Salt and pepper to season

- 100 Grams mixed vegetables (Butter beans, green beans, capsicum, broccoli, carrots and corn)

Preparation:

1. Turn oven on to 200 degrees Celsius (392 degrees Fahrenheit).

2. Combine minced beef with salt, pepper, turmeric, cinnamon, chopped onions and chives.

3. Spread and flatten the mixture onto an oven tray.

4. Add the vegetables next to the meat.

5. Bake in the oven for 45 minutes or until the meat is cooked.

6. Serve on a dish.

6   Daily Intakes

What you should try to eat on a daily basis

A balanced diet should provide your body with the right amount of nutrients to keep it healthy. This means that there are certain foods that need to be consumed on a daily basis. Whether a person's intention is to maintain weight or to lose weight, the body will still need certain nutrients to keep it healthy. The nutrients the body needs can be organized in a way that results in a calorie deficit but maximises nutrient intake.

Among the food groups that should be included in a daily nutritional plan are vegetables. Vegetables are low in calories but high in nutrients that can be good for cardiovascular health, help in preventing certain types of cancer and assist in regulating blood sugar levels. It is important to incorporate a variety of vegetables into one's diet because no single vegetable can provide all the nutrients needed for physical health.

Non-starchy vegetables such as leafy vegetables and vegetables such as broccoli and cauliflower are very low in calories and therefore can be consumed in large quantities without worrying too much about excess calories.

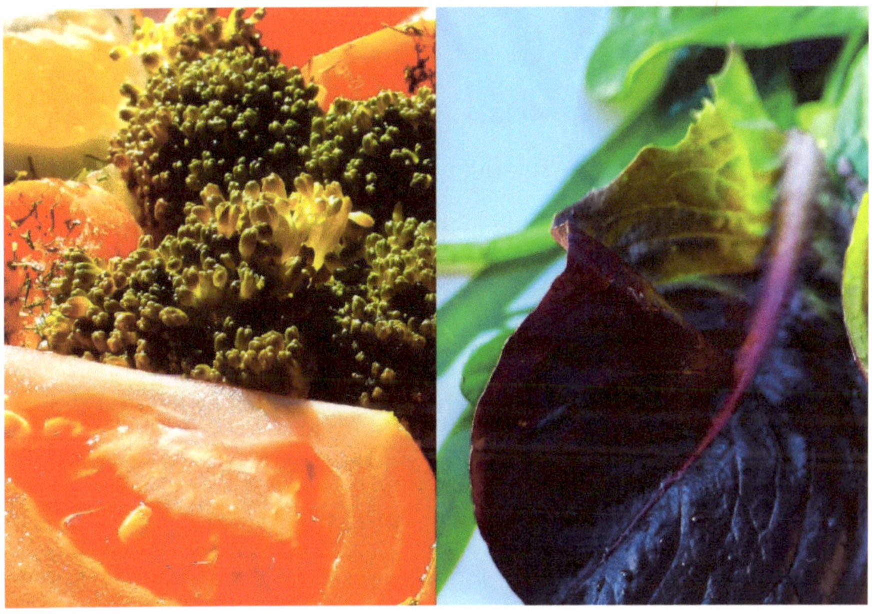

Fruits and berries can also provide vital vitamins needed for a healthy eating plan. Many berries such as blueberries and raspberries can provide antioxidants that assist the body to keep physically healthy and looking good.

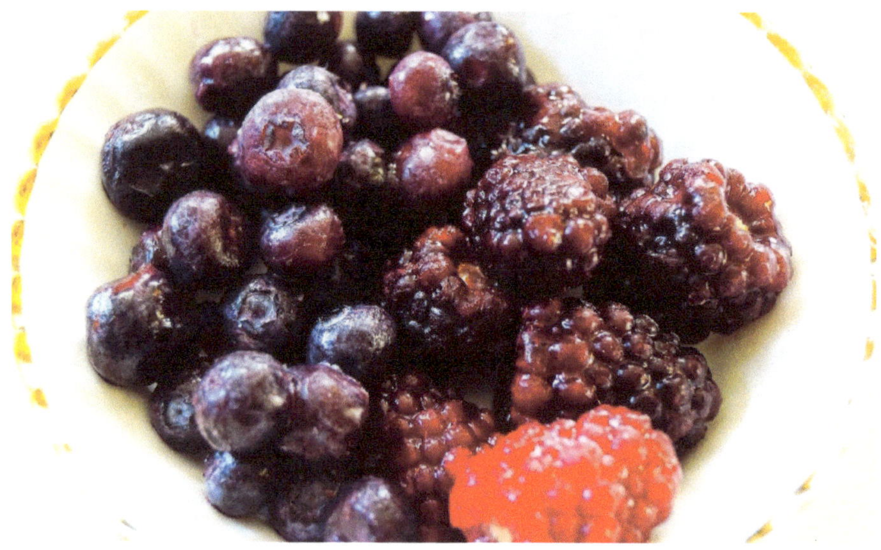

In comparison to ingredients such as nuts, legumes, meats and dairy, most fruits are relatively lower in calories per volume. However, a person can easily lose count of their calorie intake with excessive consumption of fruits, especially when added to other ingredients. Many fruits are also high in fructose and can increase blood sugar levels. So it is important to keep track of fruit intake.

A balanced diet should also include the right amount of protein. Protein is used by the body for a variety of purposes such as muscle building and tissue repair, liquid regulation and for the body's metabolic function, and for transporting and storing nutrients. The best source of protein for human beings is from animal products such as meat and dairy. Seeds (peanuts, cashews, etc.) and legumes (such as chickpeas) can also be a source of protein but individually they are usually not what are called "complete proteins". That means they do not contain all the amino acids that the human body needs to use for its protein needs. So if a person has a plant-based diet, they must insure they are eating a variety of plant-based protein sources to achieve the same benefits as a diet that includes animal products.

An important part of staying healthy while maintaining the desired weight is to keep the body hydrated.   By drinking the right amount and kinds of liquid, a person can feel satiated without adding extra calories to their daily requirements.

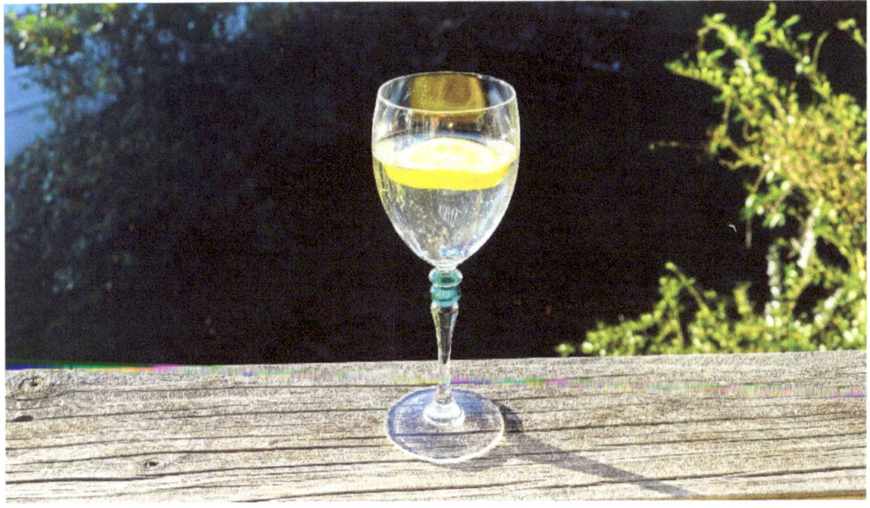

But it is important not to confuse keeping hydrated with being on a liquid diet. In fact, liquid diets in many cases are detrimental to maintaining or losing weight. Take for example the eating of a regular sized apple which when cut into pieces can fill a cup. Eating one apple can make a person feel quite satiated. However, that one apple does not provide a cup of apple juice. For a cup of pure apple juice, at least three apples need to be juiced which equals to three times the amount of calorie intake. Therefore, it is better to eat most foods in its solid form if the intention is to maintain or lose weight.

Water is one of the most essential substances needed for life so it is no wonder that adequate levels of water intake are necessary for physical health. The other benefit of drinking adequate levels of water is that it fills up the stomach and keeps an individual feeling less hungry.

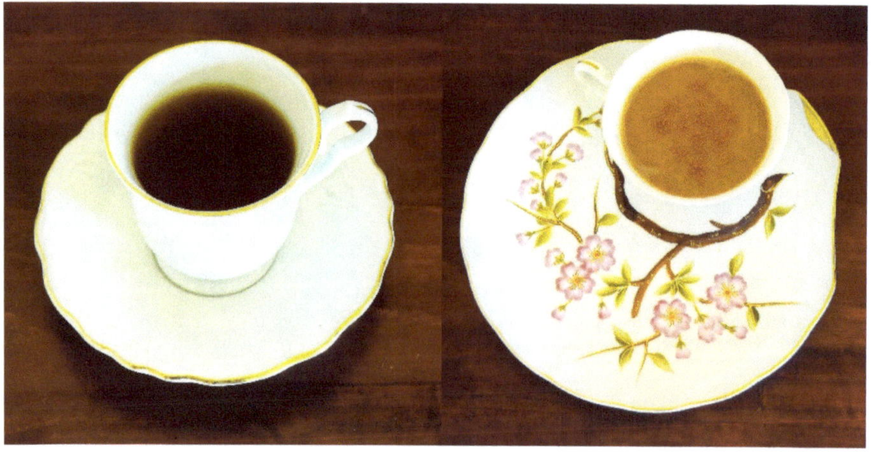

Regular black tea (nothing added): ~ 1 nutritional calorie

Cocoa and cinnamon tea with skim milk: ~ 13 nutritional calories

Ingredients: 1 Teaspoon cocoa powder, ¼ teaspoon cinnamon, 30 millilitres of trim milk

Serving size: 1 Cup

Among other drinks that are low in calories and which could be consumed on a regular basis is tea. If nothing else is added to tea, then by itself tea, like water, has almost no calories and can be a source to keep the body hydrated. Sometimes, tea can be flavoured to make it tastier by adding things such as cinnamon or cocoa. Cocoa flavoured milk tea with cinnamon is a tasty treat. The addition of other ingredients however, does add extra calories to tea that needs to be considered when calculating daily calorie consumption.

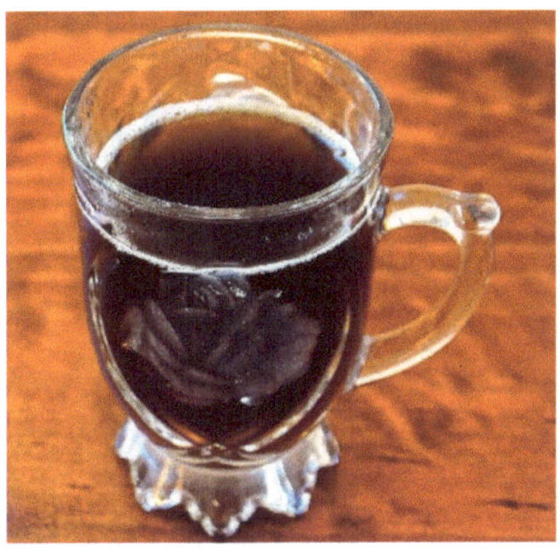

If you are a person who likes to drink tea and coffee in large quantities on a daily basis it is best to divide the added dairy to be used between all the cups consumed. Take for example, someone who drinks seven cups of tea during the day. As part of their calorie count they have incorporated 200 millilitres of daily milk intake. To ensure that the daily calorie intake is not exceeded the 200 millilitres of milk should be divided between the seven cups of tea.

A final thought to consider with regards to healthy habits is the issue of alcoholic drinks. Alcoholic drinks contain calories and drinks such as a bottle of beer are high in calories. In addition to other detrimental effects on a person's physical health, alcohol can be a major contributor to weight gain over time. So it is best for a person to reconsider their drinking habits when it comes to alcoholic drinks. Removing alcohol altogether is probably the best practice for physical and mental wellbeing.

7   Cheat Meals

How to organise a cheat meal

What is commonly referred to as a cheat meal refers to a dish that a person eats but which is usually avoided as part of their diet plan. This usually involves picking a day of the week (known as a cheat day), consuming meals or desserts that are high in calories. The idea behind the cheat meal is that if a person rewards themselves with a "treat" they enjoy for keeping to a diet, they are more likely to keep to that diet in the long term. However, there seems to be confusion among many individuals about how to integrate a cheat meal into a diet plan.

Having a cheat meal should not be about splurging on unhealthy foods or consuming large amounts of excess calories. Such a practice would be counterproductive to maintaining a healthy weight and staying physically in shape. This is because if a person eats at maintenance level of calories during the week only to consume large amounts of excess calories on one of the days of the week, they will still be consuming in excess to what their body needs to function. It was mentioned in the introduction that if the body receives calories in excess of what it needs to maintain itself, it will store the rest as excess fat weight.

The psychological aspect of cheat meals can also be detrimental rather than beneficial to staying healthy and maintaining weight. Regarding unhealthy, high calorie foods, as a treat gives the idea that healthy low calorie foods are burdensome or distasteful. But if a person is going to change their lifestyle to a healthier one, it will require them to change their habits and tastes. As mentioned in the introduction changing one's taste is an important factor to becoming accustomed to a healthier diet.

It is possible to fit in a cheat meal into a diet plan without exceeding overall calorie intake. However, in order to integrate a cheat meal into a healthy diet that maintains weight some important points should be considered. First, a cheat meal should not be treated as a reward for healthy eating. The reward is the health benefits and for some the aesthetic results of eating healthy.

But each individual might want to enjoy a particular favourite food once in a while which they would not ordinarily have as part of their diet plan. To do this they have to make sure that having that cheat meal does not add excess calories to their overall calorie intake during the week. This can be done by eating a little less than maintenance calorie level during the week and making up for it with a cheat meal that is higher in calories and makes up for the weekly calorie deficit. Another way to have a cheat meal is by leaving a day aside where during that day other parts of a person's diet is not consumed and replaced with what would be equivalent in calories to the cheat meal.

It would probably be beneficial to prepare a cheat meal that is still made up of healthy ingredients. On the following page you can find one idea of a cheat meal that is made of healthy ingredients.

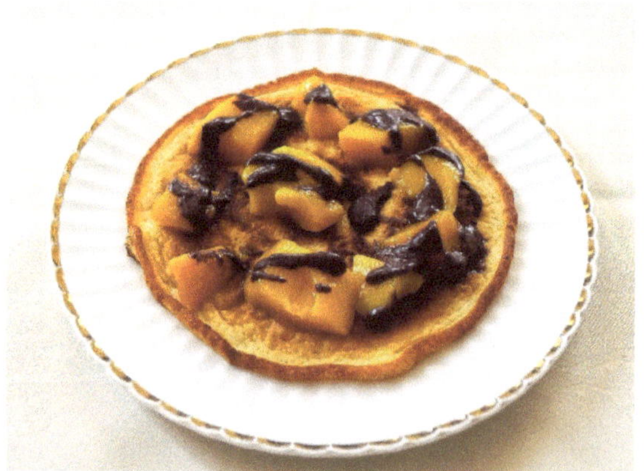

Low Calorie Pancake

Calories: ~341 (nutritional calories)

Serving: 1 Person

Ingredients:

- 2 Tablespoons self-rising flour

- 1 Chicken egg

- 200 Millilitres of skim milk

- 50 Grams frozen or fresh mangoes

- 10 Grams 90% dark chocolate (the chocolate used in this recipe is 119 calories for 20 grams)

Preparation:

1. In a bowl, combine the egg, milk and self-rising flour.

2. Blend the mixture (either by hand or a hand blender) until it is a smooth consistency.

3. Pour the mixture into a pan and let it cook until you see small bubbles forming on the top of the pancake and the mixture has cooked through.

4. Flip over the pancake to cook the other side until golden.

5. Melt the dark chocolate in a small pot.

6. Place the mangoes on the pancake.

7. Drizzle the pancake with the dark chocolate.